Intensive Care Infections

APR Wilson
Senior Lecturer in Microbiology
Department of Clinical Microbiology
University College Hospital
Grafton Way
London, UK

MARTIN DUNITZ

First published in the United Kingdom
in 1996 by
Martin Dunitz Ltd
The Livery House
7–9 Pratt Street
London NW1 0AE

A CIP record for this book is available from the British Library.

ISBN 1-85317-339-8

Printed and bound in Spain by Cayfosa

Contents

Introduction

The management of infection in the critically ill patient requires close co-operation between colleagues from many specialities. Some patients will require treatment of severe community acquired infection but many more develop nosocomial infections as the result of endotracheal intubation, catheterization, invasive monitoring, parenteral therapy and immune suppression. Most patients in the intensive care unit receive broad spectrum antibiotics, encouraging the emergence of resistant pathogens. The open design of most units, pressure of work, the dependence of the patients and the large numbers of staff ensure that many longer stay patients develop repeated episodes of infections which are often difficult to treat.

Colonization and cross infection

Nosocomial infection can derive from the patients own flora or from the environment, usually on the hands of attendants. At least half the infections are endogenous on which control of infection techniques would make little impact. However, most exogenous infections arise from procedures and derive from staff members.

In a European survey of 1005 intensive care units, the mean number of beds per unit was 6.6 with a mean of 4.4 nurses and 0.35 doctors per bed.[1] Only 38% of units complied with recommendations to prevent nosocomial pneumonia, namely, perioperative chest physiotherapy, use of gloves and sterile catheter for suctioning and change of breathing circuit every 48 hours (unless protected by filters). Changing of the intravenous giving set every 48 hours for clear fluid, every 24 hours for parenteral nutrition and every infusion for blood was performed by 44% of units. Finally, 51% of units had written guidelines for urinary catheter insertion and care and use (with little or no abuse) of a closed drainage system.

Handwashing is the single most important manoeuvre in the prevention of infection in the intensive care unit (ICU).

Handwashing

- Sleeves rolled above elbow, remove wristwatch
- Wet hands in running hot water, place 5ml disinfectant into palm
- Hold hands down
- Lather all parts of hand including finger tips and webs
- Rinse well, turn off taps using elbow on elbow taps and dry with paper towel

Many publications show enforcement of hygiene leads to a reduction of nosocomial infections. Chlorhexidine or povidone iodine should be used before and after an aseptic technique, before contact with a susceptible patient, after contact with body secretions or excreta or contaminated equipment, and before and after visiting patients in isolation. Hand cream should be for the individual staff member.

Good practice often succumbs to staff shortage, inadequate provision of sinks, failure to realize the importance of infection control and poor compliance by medical staff. The wearing of a wristwatch during clinical work prevents proper hand washing and should be strongly discouraged. If a single nurse is expected to care for two critically ill patients, cross infection is almost inevitable.

Source isolation, terminal disinfection, the use of disposable gloves for all body substance contacts and encouragement of hand washing has been reported to terminate an outbreak of pseudomonas pneumonia. Another outbreak was traced to the hands of one nurse providing care for three affected patients, the strain isolated from each being indistinguishable. In one survey, 82% of nurses were allocated to one patient but 71% assisted with procedures on other patients. Hand washing was performed after only 74% of endotracheal suction, 52% of mouth care procedures and 24% of urinary catheter bag emptying.[2]

Doctors cannot be exempt from infection control and can easily spread pathogens to any of the patients in the unit. The hands of doctors have higher bacterial counts and carriage of *Staphylococcus aureus* than nursing staff, 36% compared with 18% in one study.[3] Nurses are more frequently transient hand carriers of Gram negative bacteria. The doctor is less likely to wash his hands than the nurse or other staff except radiographers (Figure 1).[4] Consultants washed even less often than junior doctors (before 4% versus 18%; after 22% versus 26%). Contrary to expectations, staff members are more likely to wash hands after using gloves for a procedure than if gloves are not used (141/261, 54% versus 494/1207, 41%).[4]

Clearly the importance of hand washing is not sufficiently understood. Infection control education and feedback of infection rates to medical staff will help raise awareness. Antiseptic hand washing will reduce colonization, judged by fingertip cultures on agar, to very low levels. The use of non sterile clean latex gloves over washed or unwashed hands achieves a similar low count. Unfortunately any benefit is lost if the gloves are not changed or washed before touching another patient.

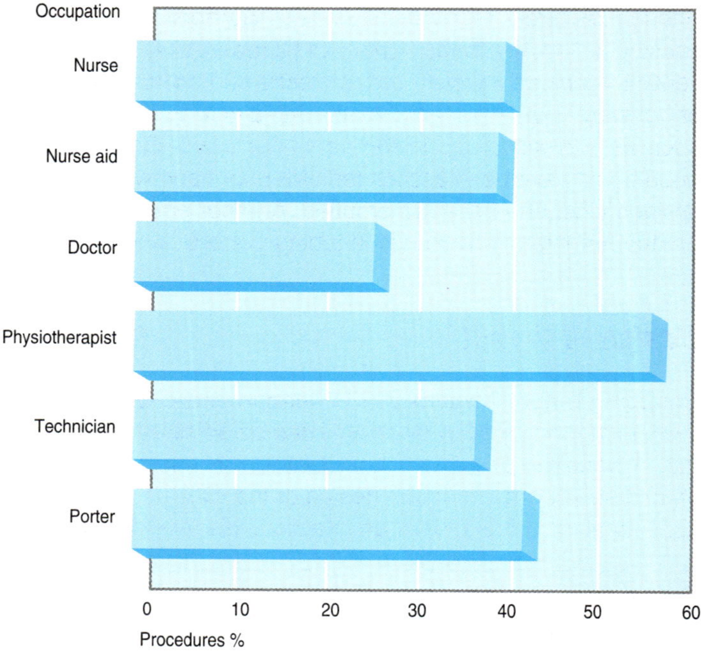

Figure 1
Proportion of contacts with patient followed by hand washing in different groups.[4]

In comparison with hand carriage, infection by the airborne route is rare, and expensive filtered air provides little additional benefit.

The most common pathogens in the ICU are:

- *Pseudomonas aeruginosa*
- *Escherichia coli*
- *Klebsiella* spp
- *Candida* spp
- enterococci

These are rarely recovered from air. Spread of pathogens causing nosocomial pneumonia can be reduced by filters in the ventilator tubing that retain both moisture and bacteria. The use of hot water humidifiers allows the rapid growth of organisms such as *Klebsiella* spp in the ventilator traps. Outbreaks of pneumonia have been associated with poor hand washing and spillage when the traps are emptied. Another potential source are the quivers in which suction tubing is stored between use.

Design of the ICU

Enforcing proper hygiene in old, inappropriate wards never intended for occupation by an ICU can be difficult and frustrating. Whenever possible, expert advice in infection control should be sought during the design of the ICU, usually from a consultant microbiologist or an infectious disease physician.[5]

Guidelines for ICU designs

- Controlled access with no through traffic allowed
- Clean and dirty utility rooms separate
- Flooring seamless to ease cleaning
- Air conditioning with appropriate filters giving ≥ 6 air changes / room / hour and in side rooms switchable between exhaust and plenum to allow for protective and source isolation
- Sinks for hand washing with hot and cold mixing faucets that can be operated by elbow and within easy access of each bed (between each 2 beds) and in every side room
- Side rooms available for source isolation, ideally with two doors and an anteroom (20 square feet, 1.8 m^2) with a sink, with a means of storage of gloves, plastic aprons and doctors' coats at the door
- Beds must be well spaced to allow movement of staff and bulky equipment and to discourage staff passing rapidly from one patient to the next without hand washing
- It has been recommended that there should be a minimum floor area per bed of 225 square feet (21 m^2) or 250 square feet (23 m^2) for a side room[5]

Unfortunately, custom made design is not a guaranteed method of reducing nosocomial infection. Huebner et al found an infection rate of 34.2% in a 65 year old converted ward and 31.9% after moving to a new unit with increased provision of side rooms.[6] A fall in the incidence of pneumonia (16%–12%) was ascribed to improvements in respiratory equipment and a control study rather than improved design.

Investigation and management of outbreaks

For some infections, isolation of the patient is necessary to prevent spread within the unit. Source isolation is used particularly for patients with:

- diarrhoea and vomiting
- rash and fever
- new suspected open tuberculosis
- suspected streptococcal cellulitis
- previous known carriage of resistant pathogens such as methicillin resistant *Staphylococcus aureus* (MRSA), aminoglycoside resistant coliforms and vancomycin resistant *Enterococcus faecalis* (VRE)

Source isolation

- Remove white coat, wash and dry hands, put on gloves and plastic apron
- Enter room, complete task, dispose of contaminated items in colour coded bags and needles in sharps bin
- Dispose of gloves and apron into colour coded bag
- Wash and dry hands, leave room, wash hands again. Keep door closed

In contrast, protective isolation is used to prevent infection of an immunocompromised patient by staff, visitors or the environment. The procedure is similar except that gloves and apron are removed outside the room.

Two or more cases of a particular infection in one area defines an outbreak. It is only possible to show that two isolates of the same species are indistinguishable not that they are the same. The cases must be recorded with the time of onset of symptoms and the Infection Control Nurse or Officer should be informed. Specimens must be collected for culture and the cases put in source isolation. If sufficient side rooms are not available, it may be possible to restrict cases to a particular bay and to provide cohort nursing to minimize spread. Patients with different strains of MRSA can be nursed together. It may be difficult to restrict the movement of unaffected patients from an ICU but they should stay in side rooms on the receiving ward until cultures are negative. The microbiologist may need to screen other patients and the staff. If cases continue to be identified, the temporary closure of part or all of the unit will have to be considered.

MRSA

Staphylococcus aureus resistant to methicillin (flucloxacillin, nafcillin) is usually resistant to many other antibiotics and is mediated by a change in the penicillin binding proteins which have a low affinity for penicillins and cephalosporins. Treatment with vancomycin or teicoplanin is expensive. Individual clinicians may not appreciate an increase in clinically serious infections and antibiotic costs in the whole hospital and may disregard repeated advice to wash hands. The importance of MRSA is largely as a marker of cross infection. It is not clearly more pathogenic than methicillin sensitive strains but colonization may be more likely to result in significant disease. Carriage makes discharge from the unit or the hospital (except to home) more difficult. The organism is frequently imported into hospitals when colonized patients or their household contacts are readmitted. Staff members may unwittingly disseminate the organism around the other patients and screening may be needed.

Action on finding MRSA carrier

- The patient must be source isolated, movement in the hospital restricted and the notes marked
- Any surgery must be performed at the end of a session
- Other carriage sites (nose, hairline, groin, axilla) should be screened
- Other patients with wounds on the unit should be screened
- If another patient is found to carry a similar strain, screening of the staff and remaining patients should be performed

In carriers without open wounds, eradication of the organism may be attempted and, with source isolation, is effective in terminating outbreaks. Antiseptic shampoo and skin cleanser (chlorhexidine) and nasal ointment (mupirocin) are used for five days. The patient can be released from isolation only after three negative screens separated by 3–7 days. Staff carriers may return to work once they have applied topical antiseptics for two days. After discharge of patients from source isolation, surfaces should be wiped with a phenolic in addition to the usual cleaning. Even in units where MRSA is endemic, intensive surveillance, cohort nursing of colonized patients (separating infected patients and their carers from other patients), eradication protocols, and source isolation are effective if sufficient resources are made available.

Vancomycin resistant enterococci (VRE)

VRE are far less common than MRSA but are usually resistant to all commonly available antibiotics and can cause an untreatable septicaemia. Most strains possess a gene called vanA which enables the organism to produce a cell wall component less likely to bind glycopeptides. Enterococci with vanA are resistant to vancomycin and teicoplanin and can transfer this property to other enterococci and, in the laboratory, to *Staphylococcus aureus*. The less common vanB and vanC enterococci are resistant to vancomycin but usually sensitive to teicoplanin.

Prevalence is increasing throughout the USA and Europe, particularly in areas of high antibiotic use. A rise in the proportion of resistant strains from 0.4% to 13.6% was noted in ICUs in the USA over four years. Many more patients are colonized, usually in the gut, than are actually infected. In an infected ICU the rate of colonization may be between 10% and 33% depending on the form of surveillance. Colonization persists for many months. Transmission is most likely from patients with diarrhoea and contaminated rectal probes, a low air-loss bed and bedpans have been implicated in outbreaks. Oral vancomycin, given to treat pseudomembranous colitis, is a possible risk factor. Source isolation and rigorous enforcement of handwashing will slow the rate of colonization but are unlikely to be fully effective unless there is strict control of antibiotic use, particularly cephalosporins.

Aminoglycoside resistant coliforms

Multiply resistant Gram negative bacteria are selected by the use of broad spectrum antibiotics and can readily transfer resistance between strains and species by means of R-factors. Many hospitals have reported outbreaks of cross infection, *Pseudomonas* spp being associated with contaminated ECG electrodes, lumbar puncture needles or topical antibiotics. The withdrawal of ampicillin in a unit terminated one outbreak of *Klebsiella* spp. The hands of staff members remain the most important mode of spread and reinforcement of hand washing the most effective method of control (Table 1).[7]

Washing	Number of Experiments	Number showing 98% reduction in counts
Warm water	8	0
Chlorhexidine hand cleanser	23	19
Non-medicated soap	4	2
Medicated soap	13	10

Table 1
Effect of washing on counts of viable Klebsiella *spp on experimentally inoculated hands (Casewell).*[7]

Penicillin resistant pneumococci

Penicillin resistant isolates of pneumococci are becoming common in many countries. In Spain, they have increased from 37% in 1987 to 46% in 1992, and in France the prevalence is 12% Many can still be treated with large doses of penicillins but approximately 1% of strains in the USA are now highly resistant. Strains with an MIC of penicillin of ≥2 mg/l have probably acquired resistance from other species and are commonly resistant to chloramphenicol, erythromycin and clindamycin. Outbreaks occur in the community particularly amongst children but there is a risk of spread within the ICU and source isolation is advisable. Cephalosporins are a common choice for treatment of these infections but failure of treatment has been reported with pneumococci resistant to ceftriaxone. Glycopeptides are an alternative treatment in areas of high resistance.

Diagnosis and management of infection

Diagnosis of nosocomial infection can be difficult, particularly in the surgical or trauma patient. Fever and leucocytosis are often present in both infected and uninfected patients and the C-reactive protein remains high for some weeks after major surgery. Using 'clinical evaluation' as the gold standard, Fassbender et al[8] found that a fever over 38°C identified the 13 infected patients in a population of 104 with a sensitivity of 54% and specificity of 90%. The cytokine, IL-6, a mediator of the inflammatory response, was a highly specific indicator though less sensitive than C-reactive protein (Table 2). However, assay is expensive.

There are few prospective controlled trials of antibiotic use in ICU and most dogma is derived from small uncontrolled trials. In evaluating the standard of management of infection, some method of case control is necessary by age, diagnosis, severity of illness and prior length of stay in the ICU. The various commonly used scoring methods such as APACHE II or SAPS, are helpful but not specific to infection.

Parameter	Sensitivity	Specificity	Positive predictive value	Negative predictive value
C-reactive protein <>130mg/L	85	83	69	97
IL-6 <> 35 pg/mL	69	97	82	94

Table 2
Comparison of CRP and IL–6 as diagnostic indicators of nosocomial infection (13 infected patients in 104).[8]

Nosocomial versus community acquired infections

Infection is considered to be nosocomial when it develops more than 72 hours after hospital admission. Patients in the ICU are at high risk of infection and the ICU is commonly the source of infections spreading to other wards. Pneumonia, urinary infection, bacteraemia and wound infection are common, the rate of infection being correlated with the length of stay and highest in relation to invasive devices. Of 170 patients admitted to one ICU, 83 developed a documented infection and a systemic inflammatory response, and 12 septic shock.[9]

Pneumonia

Of 8361 patients in European ICUs, 10% had pneumonia on admission and another 11% developed pneumonia during their stay.[1] The mortality rate was 31%. There was some variation between countries, probably reflecting the selection of patients for intensive care (Figure 2). Of these patients, 29% had microbiological evidence in addition to clinical signs. Significant risk factors were APACHE II score over seven, ventilation for at least two days, sedation, surgery and shock. In the USA,

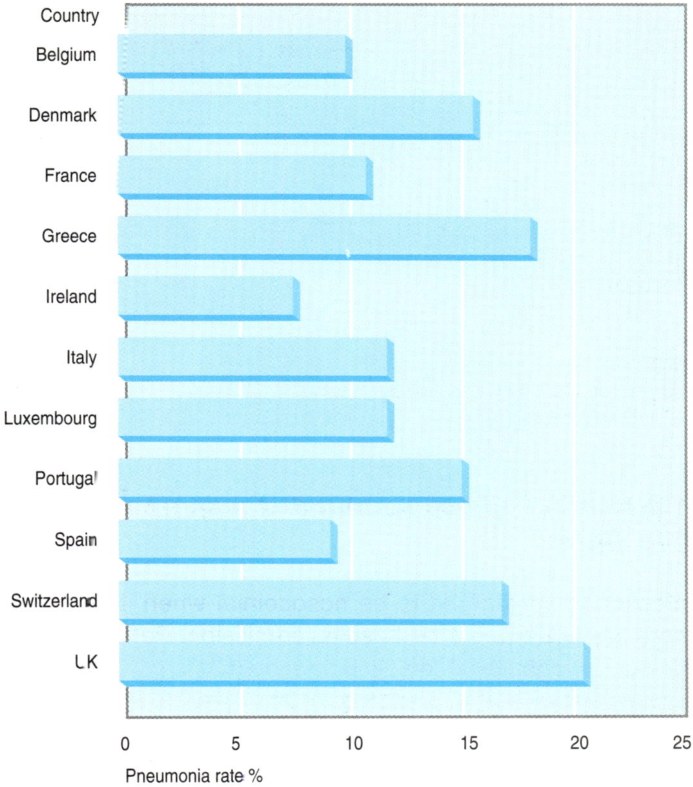

Figure 2
Prevalence of pneumonia in European ICUs.[1]

20–60% of ventilated patients develop pneumonia with a mean additional hospital stay of 10 days. Pneumonia is the cause of 12–21% of cases of the Adult Respiratory Distress Syndrome (ARDS) when it is associated with a mortality of 67%.[10] Pneumonia can develop secondary to ARDS. Generalized damage to the micro circulation allows exudation of fluid into the alveoli preventing clearance of bacteria and impairing the action of inflammatory cells.

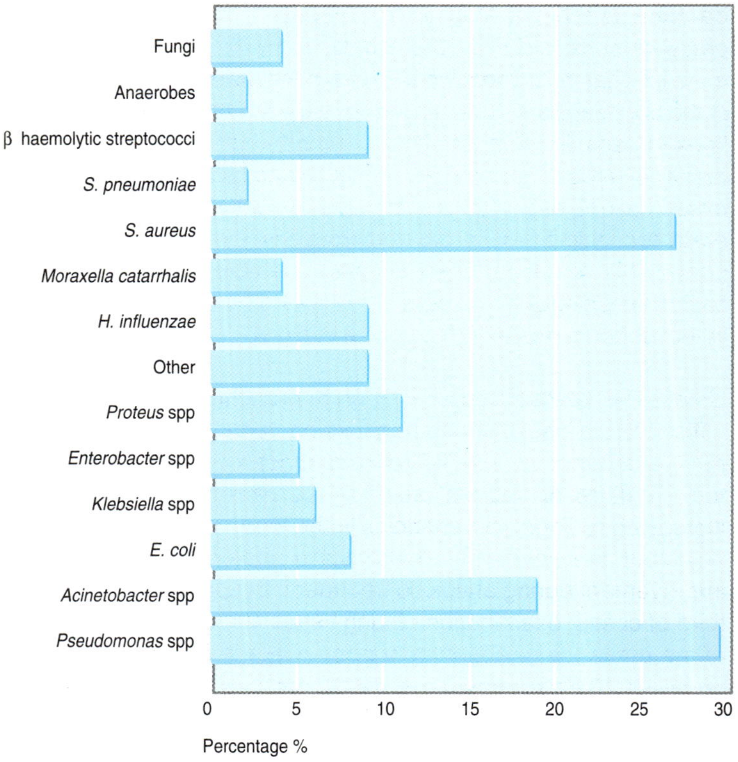

Figure 3
Bacterial isolates in ventilator associated pneumonia. Pooled results of 115 episodes.[11]

Ventilated patients, particularly those receiving antibiotics, soon become colonized in the oropharynx, sinuses and trachea by aerobic Gram negative bacteria, the usual causes of nosocomial pneumonia (Figure 3). These organisms probably originate in the upper gastrointestinal tract, plaque and gingiva. Loss of the normal flora, α-haemolytic streptococci, to antibiotic treatment encourages their proliferation. Endotracheal intubation compromises the normal protective mechanisms of the glottis and the cuff may fail to protect the lower airway from the aspiration of bacteria laden pharyngeal secretions. Large volume low pressure cuffs fold in on themselves in the trachea forming a route for pharyngeal secretions to reach the lower tract. Changes in the tracheal diameter during respiration may also allow secretions to pass. In the normal host, aspirated pharyngeal flora is rapidly cleared by mucociliary transport and IgA. In the compromised patient, aspirated aerobic Gram negative bacteria proliferate too quickly to be cleared from the lower airways and pneumonia develops. In most cases, aerobic Gram negative bacteria causing pneumonia can be isolated from the oropharynx in the 72 hours preceding the onset of signs.

Unless they are isolated from blood or bronchial washings, it is difficult to distinguish Gram negative bacteria that colonize the respiratory tract from those causing infection. Fever, leucocytosis, culture of tracheal aspirate, purulent secretions and increasing radiographic shadows in the lungs are used in diagnosis but lack specificity. Diagnosis is often made by clinical improvement during antibiotic treatment. In approximately one third of cases, examination of lung tissue shows the diagnosis of the presence or absence of pneumonia is incorrect.[12] The presence of elastin fibres in tracheal aspirate has been found to improve specificity to 73% but they may be absent in pneumococcal or mycoplasma pneumonia.[13]

Fibreoptic bronchoscopy can be used to collect brush or lavage specimens from the lower airways free of contamination from pharyngeal flora. Bronchoalveolar lavage (BAL) requires introduction of 120 ml of saline into a distal bronchus in several aliquots. A colony count in the withdrawn fluid of 10^4 cfu/ml is diagnostic but patients with bronchitis can reach these counts without pneumonia. Mixed cultures, which are common in nosocomial pneumonia, may be considered negative if individual species are less than 10^4 cfu/ml.[12] A Gram stain of the fluid is valuable in showing the bacteria, elastin fibres and neutrophils that are more common in pneumonia. In various small series using histological criteria, sensitivity of BAL is between 72% and 100% and specificity is between 66% and 100%.[14]

Hypoxia, worsening of infiltrates and fever are potential complications. In one series of 27 patients without any signs of infection, 4 had lavage counts of >10^5 cfu/ml. Lavage without bronchoscopy can give a sensitivity of 73% and specificity of 96% but experience is more limited.[15] Protected brush specimens have good sensitivity and specificity as the brush is not exposed to pharyngeal secretions and is advanced under direct vision into bronchial pus. The presence of 1000 cfu/ml ($\equiv 1 \times 10^6$ cfu/ml in bronchi) is diagnostic. A sensitivity of 100% and specificity of 60% has been reported for the procedure sampling lung tissue from ventilated patients soon after death but sensitivity falls to 13% if antibiotics have been given.[12] Some hypoxaemic patients may not be able to tolerate the procedure and a false negative result can lead to needed therapy being withheld.

Bacteria may be inhaled as an aerosol, seeded in the lung during bacteraemia or spread from an empyema. Aspiration of gastric contents is a common reason for admission to the ICU and infection may develop with anaerobic and upper respiratory flora. The stomach can become colonized with aerobic Gram negative bacteria during ileus or use of H_2 blockers and act as a reservoir. Bacterial overgrowth can be prevented by maintaining gastric acidity while protecting the gastric mucosa with an agent such as sucralfate. Controlled trials suggest no significant difference in the incidence of pneumonia in patients given either sucralfate or ranitidine. Enteral feeding reduces the efficacy of sucralfate or topical antibiotics in reducing colonization of the stomach by bacteria.[12] Sinusitis is another significant risk factor for the development of pneumonia and might be associated with the use of nasogastric tubes. In contrast to community acquired sinusitis which is caused by pneumococci and *Haemophilus influenzae*, nosocomial sinusitis is caused by mixed Gram negative flora.

Heat and moisture exchanging filters reduce loss of heat and moisture during expiration and are a barrier to bacteria. They protect the patient from bacterial or viral pathogens in the ventilator and protect the ventilator from contamination by the patient's flora. The efficiency of hygroscopic–hydrophobic filters seems similar to that of hydrophobic filters but the former allow better humidification. If bacterial filters are not used, condensation quickly promotes bacterial growth in the circuit to levels of $2x10^5$ cfu/ml yet changing the circuit every 48 hours does not reduce the incidence of pneumonia. Heated water humidifier systems are effective but there is a risk of formation of a bacterial aerosol.

Pneumonia caused by *Staphylococcus aureus* is a particular risk in the patients with tricuspid endocarditis, secondary to drug abuse, and in ventilated neurosurgical patients. The latter probably aspirate the organisms in upper respiratory secretions during the initial trauma or surgery.

Community acquired pneumonia is less common in the ICU and is most often caused by infection with *Streptococcus pneumoniae*. The frequency of other pathogens varies according to the population surveyed:

- *Haemophilus influenzae*
- *Legionella* spp
- *Chlamydia* spp
- *Mycoplasma* spp
- *Staphylococcus aureus*
- Gram negative bacteria

Of a series of 299 patients with community acquired pneumonia admitted to an ICU, the causative organism was isolated in 197 (66%): *Streptococcus pneumoniae* (31%), *Staphylococcus* spp (22%), and *Haemophilus influenzae* (10%). *S. pneumoniae* was present with other pathogens in another 29 (14%) cases.[16] In only 3% was *Pseudomonas aeruginosa* implicated. Blood cultures were positive in 46 patients, *S. pneumoniae* being the usual isolate.

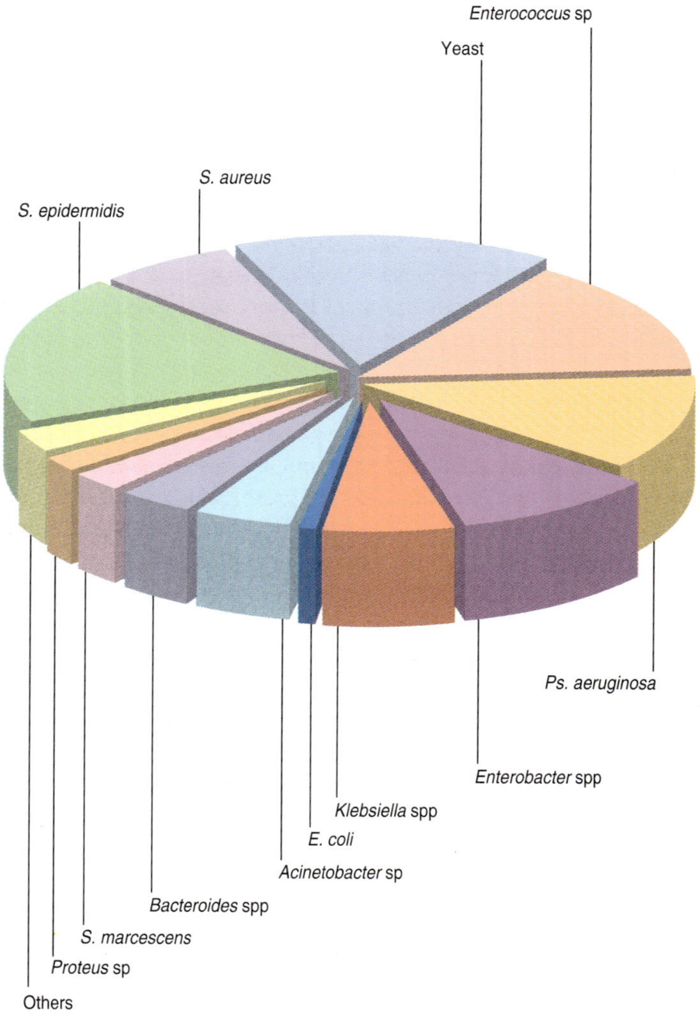

Figure 4
Causative organisms in 300 surgical patients with septic shock.[17]

Septicaemia and septic shock

The sepsis (or septic) syndrome can be caused by overwhelming infection by Gram positive or Gram negative bacteria, fungi, parasites or viruses (Figure 4).[17] Blood stream infection caused by *Escherichia coli, Streptococcus pneumoniae* and coagulase negative staphylococci have the highest survival rates, those with *Pseudomonas aeruginosa* and fungi the worst, possibly because of their resistance to many agents.[18] Sepsis from the urinary tract is more likely to respond to treatment and has a greater survival than that from the respiratory or gastrointestinal tracts (Figure 5).[18,19]

There are no clinical factors that will reliably predict bacteraemia in clinically septic surgical patients but 40% of such patients will have respiratory, urinary, venous catheter or wound infections. Translocation of endotoxin or bacteria from the gastrointestinal tract can occur in severe stress such as major burns. Fever, drug abuse, rigors, severe underlying illness, hypotension and abdominal pain are helpful predictors. All body fluids should be cultured in addition to investigation by radiography, ultrasound or surgery if appropriate.

Patients may develop acidosis, disseminated intravascular coagulation, organ ischaemia, pulmonary oedema and end organ damage. Signs are neither sensitive nor specific nor does their severity necessarily relate to the severity of the syndrome. The term systemic inflammatory response syndrome (SIRS) has now been proposed to cover the presentation which can arise from both infectious causes and trauma, burns or other insults.[20] SIRS is sensitive but needs to be used with a severity of illness score.

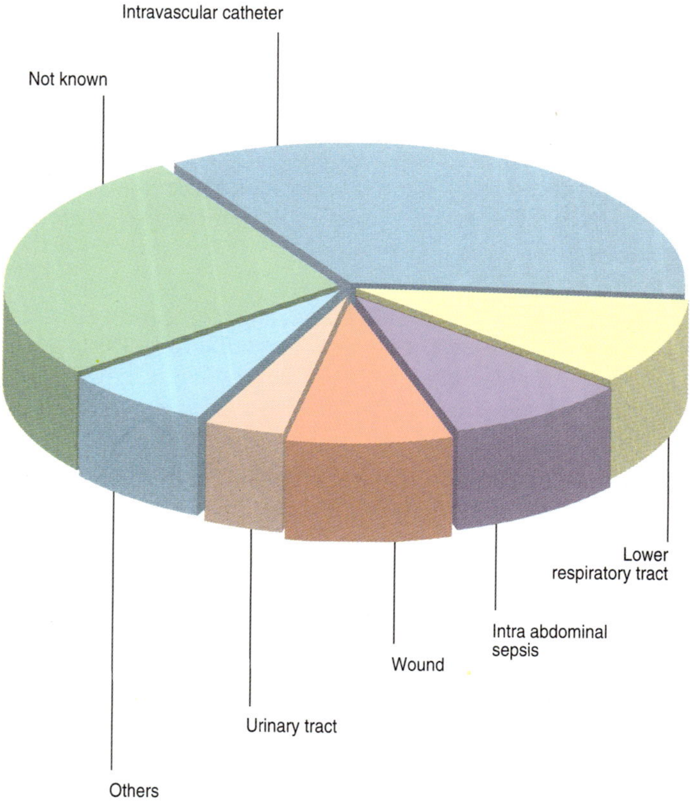

Figure 5
Site of infection in 111 ICU patients.[19]

The sepsis syndrome:[20]

- Clinical evidence of infection
- Fever or hypothermia (>38.3°C or <35.6°C)
- Tachypnoea (>20/min or ventilated)
- Tachycardia (>90/min)
- Impaired organ system function or perfusion: systolic blood pressure <90mmHg or two of: confusion, arterial hypoxaemia, unexplained metabolic acidosis, oliguria, reduction platelets/abnormal clotting, increased cardiac output/low peripheral resistance

SIRS

Patients have two or more of: body temperature >38°C or <36°C, heart rate >90/min, respiratory rate >20/min or $PaCO_2$ <4.3 kPa, and white cell count $>12x10^9/l$ or $<4x10^9/l$ or >10% band forms.

In a series of 300 surgical patients with shock, 215 (72%) died.[17] If three or more organs fail, death is inevitable. Most studies find that poor antimicrobial treatment, severe underlying disease and multi-organ failure precede death. Scoring systems, such as APACHE III, applied to patients who did and did not meet sepsis syndrome criteria produce overlapping mortality risks in both groups. Changes in the weightings used for some risk factors have been proposed which improve the predictive power of APACHE in sepsis.[21]

Sepsis syndrome can be reproduced in animal models by the injection of endotoxin, the lipopolysaccaride of the cell wall of Gram negative bacteria, or the teichoic acid of Gram positive bacteria. The response is mediated by cytokines such as tumour necrosis factor, interleukin 1, interleukin 6, and interleukin 8 released by macrophages. They act on neutrophil leucocytes promoting phagocytosis and killing of bacteria by production of free oxygen radicals, elastase and collagenase. The enzyme superoxide dismutase normally ensures that this process occurs only at the site of infection. If the patient is shocked, release of free radicals occurs throughout the body damaging connective tissue and leading to multiple organ failure.

Tumour necrosis factor (TNF) will also reproduce the signs of endotoxaemia when injected into animals. It is released in response to a wide variety of organisms including staphylococci and influenza virus and plasma levels are usually correlated with mortality. TNF is damaging when large quantities are released but in animals smaller quantities can be protective. TNF stimulates endothelial cells to release tissue factor and platelet activating factor promoting thrombosis and it controls fibrinolysis. TNF also causes the margination and transmigration of white cells. Colony stimulating factors and interleukin-8 are released, activating and directing leucocytes. Various effects on the vasculature can be produced by the release of prostacycline I2, prostaglandin E2, thromboxane, nitric oxide and endothelin.

Another important mediator, interleukin-1, is infrequently detected in plasma (<10%). It has a short half life and may be concentrated in tissues. Studies are divided as to a correlation between plasma levels of IL-1β and mortality. Further along the inflammatory cascade, interleukin-6 remains longer in the circulation and is more easily measured. High concentrations have been related consistently to mortality.

Catheter related sepsis

Catheter related sepsis

- Insertion site infection: purulent discharge or ≥15 colony forming units (cfu) on semiquantitative culture
- Catheter infection by ≥15 cfu (or 1000 colonies on quantitative culture) from the distal part of the catheter. Colonization is present when the number of cfu is below 15
- Catheter related bacteraemia: blood and catheter cultures produce growth of an indistinguishable organism

Infection of vascular access catheters may be associated with swelling, redness, discharge and thrombophlebitis at the site but often the only sign is a fever unresponsive to empirical antibiotics. Once removed, a catheter can be cultured by rolling on an agar plate (semi-quantitative) or by sonication or flushing in broth followed by quantitative plating. The latter method identifies intraluminal as well as extraluminal infection. Coagulase negative staphylococci are the causative organisms in half catheter related bacteraemias, and a third of all bacteraemias (Figure 6),[22] another 10% are caused by *Staphylococcus aureus* and smaller numbers by coliforms or yeasts. Of 442 pulmonary artery catheters in one trial, 96 (22%) showed colonization of the catheter or sheath and five were associated with bacteraemia, all having been in situ more than five days.[23]

Thrombus and a fibrin coating can develop within 24 hours of insertion. The use of chlorhexidine/silver sulphadiazine or cephazolin bonded to the plastic has been shown to reduce the incidence of infection. Catheters with, or attached to, a number of infusion ports or stopcocks are at greater risk of infection from increased handling. Up to one half of stopcocks are expected to be contaminated and the catheter hub is the most frequent source of bacteraemia. Pressure transducers present a similar risk. There is no significant difference in the rate of infection of single or multiple lumen catheters in controlled trials and it is likely that technique of insertion and manipulation is more important. Frequently only a single lumen is in use at any one time. Change of giving sets at one, two or three day intervals has been associated with similar rates of colonization in various catheters but one retrospective study suggested that there was less risk of infection with a minimum period of 48 hours.

The most common site of insertion is subclavian but this may carry a higher risk of pneumothorax than the internal jugular site. Subclavian catheters are at less risk of colonization than jugular or femoral catheters (Figure 7).[24] A tunnelled line is preferred if prolonged use is likely. Aseptic technique suffers during emergency insertion with a consequent higher rate of infection

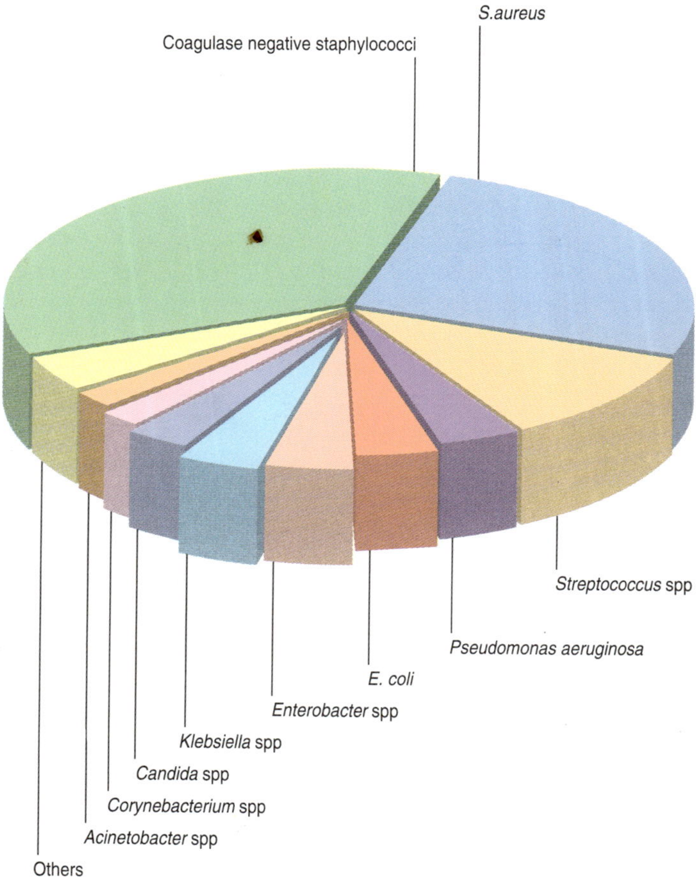

Figure 6
Clinically significant bacteraemias notified to Communicable Disease Surveillance Centre in one year.[22]

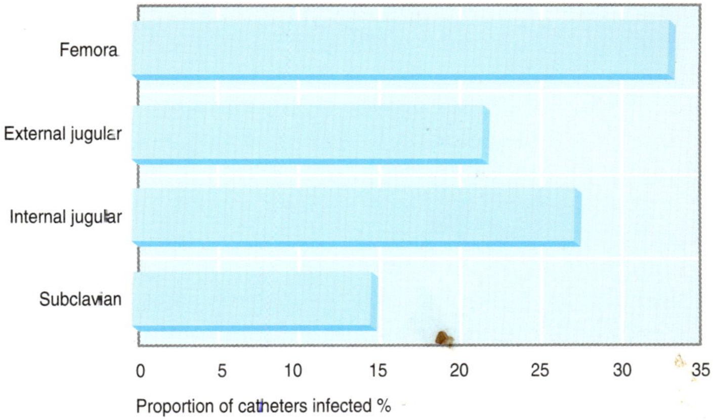

Figure 7
Proportion of catheters colonized by site of insertion.[24]

and such catheters should be exchanged after 24 hours. The best results are obtained when catheter insertion is performed in theatre using chlorhexidine or iodophor to prepare the skin. Rigorous hand washing should be carried out and sterile gloves worn. Prophylactic antibiotics do not seem to be effective and may encourage resistance.[22] A single experienced operator is preferable to a multitude of inexperienced ones. Infection rates are higher when the insertion has been found to be difficult. Gauze and film dressings for catheter exit sites are usually found to have similar rates of catheter colonization but one study reported higher rates of infection and bacteraemia with the film dressing, probably because such catheters were left in situ for longer periods.[25] New polyurethane dressings have a greater permeability to water vapour and site colonization by skin flora is less than with conventional film dressings but still greater than under gauze.[23] The use of povidone iodine at each dressing change has not been found to alter infection rates and, although mupirocin reduces colonization, its widespread use might compromise its role in clearance of carriage of MRSA.

Catheters should be removed as soon as possible if the patient has unexplained fever or positive blood cultures or if there is erythema or discharge at the insertion site or when the catheter is no longer needed. If removal is not practicable, appropriate antibiotics should be given. The longer a catheter remains in place the more likely it is to become colonized but exchange over a guidewire every 72 hours does not reduce the rate of infection nor does a change of site every week. At present, replacement in the absence of indicators of possible infection does not seem justified. Many will exchange central lines over a guidewire to preserve the site and to reduce the likelihood of complications associated with insertion. If culture of the catheter shows it to have been infected, the replacement should be removed.

Prosthetic valve endocarditis

Prosthetic valve endocarditis develops in 2–3% of patients having valve replacement (740/25 923 in one series), a third developing the infection 'early' or within 60 days of surgery (Figure 8). Coagulase negative staphylococci, Staphylococcus aureus and a-haemolytic streptococci are the common causes, the latter being usual in late infections. A paraprosthetic leak suggests a valve ring abscess. Fever, altered murmurs and

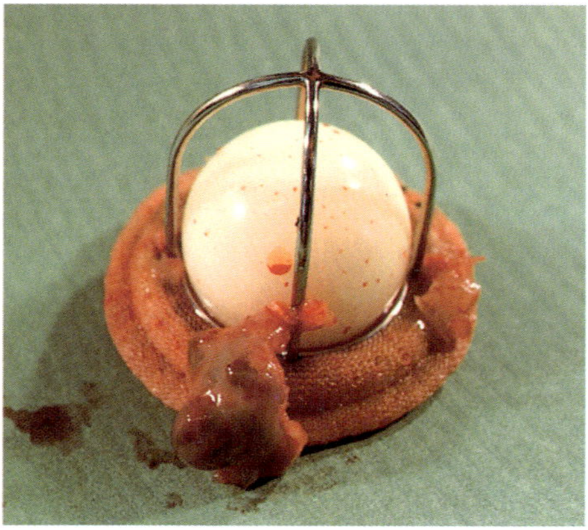

Figure 8
Vegetations on a Starr Edwards valve prosthesis.

embolic phenomena such as cerebrovascular accident, are common but other typical signs of endocarditis are often absent. Blood culture and echocardiography are essential but not always helpful. Surgery to remove the infected tissues and valve is necessary for patients with increasing heart failure, valve obstruction or leak, continued emboli or failed medical treatment. Prolonged central venous catheterization can cause life threatening native tricuspid valve endocarditis. At particular risk are patients with repeated bacteraemia, for example following major burns, or neutropenic patients in whom several episodes of catheter infection may be treated by antibiotics rather than removal of the catheter (Figure 9).

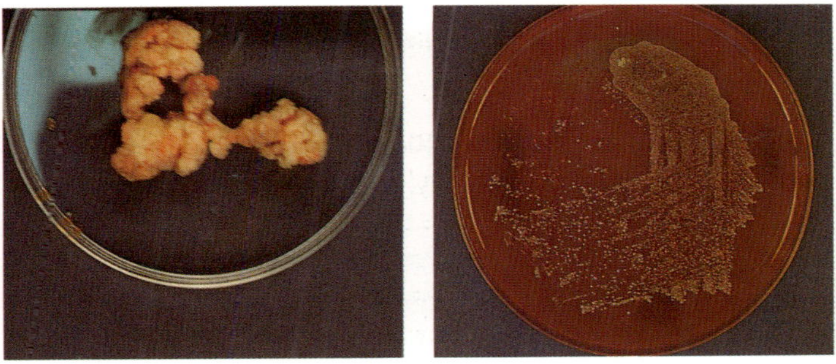

Figure 9
(a) Massive vegetation removed post mortem from a leukaemic patient caused by Hickman catheter infection; (b) Culture of the vegetation showing S.epidermidis *despite three months' treatment with high dose teicoplanin.*

Wound infection

Open wounds or burns quickly become colonized with bacteria from the patient's own flora or the environment. Erythema, serous or purulent discharge in any combination are obvious signs but fever may be the only early sign of deep seated sepsis. *Staphylococcus aureus* is most common but coagulase negative staphylococci should not be dismissed if a similar strain is repeatedly isolated from a discharging wound. *Streptococcus pyogenes* should be suspected if a superficial spreading cellulitis develops. Abdominal surgical wounds more usually become infected with a variety of Gram negative aerobes, enterococci and anaerobic bacteria. Daily dressings or debridement are sufficient in most cases, antibiotics being reserved for patients with spreading cellulitis, bacteraemia or purulent discharge with dehiscence. Irrigation with saline is effective in clearing the severe deep seated infections. Intra-abdominal sepsis may require repeated laparotomies and lavage or irrigation.

Necrotizing fasciitis occurs after abdominal surgery, ischiorectal infection or even a minor injury to a limb. It is a rapidly progressive infective necrosis of superficial and deep fascia and subcutaneous fat and carries a high mortality. *Streptococcus pyogenes* with *Bacteroides* spp and coliforms are often isolated. Progressive bacterial gangrene of the skin and fat can occur in ischaemic tissues following surgery and is caused by *Staphylococcus aureus* and microaerophilic streptococci. Shock quickly develops. Dusky purple areas within cellulitis are an early sign. Gas gangrene is a rare complication of surgical wounds caused by *Clostridium* spp and is suggested by grey discoloration around a wound with serous discharge or bullae. A high index of suspicion is important in all cases and treatment with intravenous fluids and antibiotics urgent. Excision of the necrotic tissue should be considered in an emergency.

Urinary infection

Urethral catheterization or instrumentation is the usual cause of urinary infection in the ICU. Urinary catheters inevitably become colonized with bacteria within two weeks of insertion either through the lumen if disconnected or between the catheter and urethral wall. Bacteraemia occurs in about 1% of patients. Abdominal pain, rigors, confusion or fever in a patient with a urethral catheter should be investigated by blood culture. Culture of catheter urine will only be helpful in identifying the source of an organism in the blood. Antibiotics are not necessary in the absence of symptoms and the pathogens are frequently multiply resistant Gram negative bacilli. Bacteraemia requires systemic antibiotics and removal of the catheter. A closed sterile drainage system will delay but not prevent catheter infection.

Gastrointestinal infection

Diarrhoea in the critically ill is usually due to the osmotic effect or rapid administration of enteric feeds, lactose intolerance or mucosal damage due to ischaemia. However, the stool should be cultured for *Salmonella* spp, *Shigella* spp and *Campylobacter* spp. *Vibrio cholerae* must be considered in travellers or in endemic areas. Typhoid (enteric fever) is associated with constipation rather than diarrhoea in the first week. In the second week of illness, perforation and faecal peritonitis may develop. With the exception of typhoid, supportive rather than antibiotic treatment is needed. All patients with presumed infectious diarrhoea should be kept in source isolation.

Clostridium difficile is present in the gut in up to 3% of adults, 20% of in-patients and 40% of neonates, and is a common cause of diarrhoea in the ICU. Changes in bowel flora following antibiotic therapy may allow increased growth of this organism in addition to other anaerobes. By production of toxins, pathogenic strains produce a range of disease from transient diarrhoea to pseudomembranous colitis or toxic megacolon. Diagnosis is best made by inspection and biopsy via a sigmoidoscope but many prefer to rely on laboratory demonstration of toxin in the stool. The most sensitive and specific method is observation of the cytotoxicity of toxin B in stool against tissue culture. Immunoassays are available but not as sensitive. The cephalosporins, ampicillin and clindamycin are often implicated in antibiotic associated colitis. Withdrawal of antibiotics when diarrhoea starts is adequate treatment for most cases but in the critically ill oral vancomycin will usually lead to improvement in 3 days. Metronidazole may be less effective but does not exert a selective pressure for the emergence of vancomycin resistant enterococci. If treatment fails, colectomy may be necessary. The organism is easily spread within the ICU on hands of carers so it is important to source isolate patients with diarrhoea and reinforce hand washing.

Fungal Infections

Systemic fungal infections are a common cause of death in patients with prolonged neutropenia, solid tumours, AIDS or organ transplants but diagnosis is difficult. *Candida* spp, *Aspergillus* spp, *Cryptococcus* spp and the zygomycetes and, in some areas, *Histoplasma capsulatum* and *Coccidioides immitis* can cause invasive infections (Table 3). Systemic candidal infection has been reported in 11% of patients with leukaemia, 1% of those with lymphoma and 4% of those with sarcoma (Figure 10). Patients with lung or heart lung transplants develop fungal infection in 15–35% of cases as may one fifth of patients with heart transplants (usually *Aspergillus* spp).

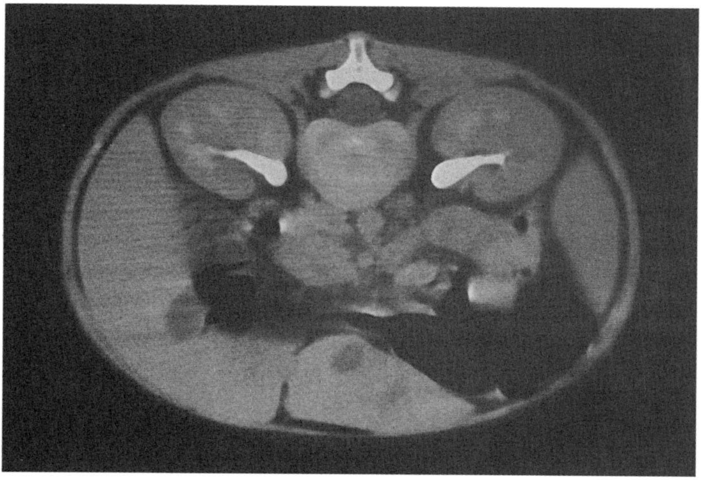

Figure 10
Hepatosplenic candidiasis in a transplant patient. CT scan of abdomen.

Pathogen	Signs and complications	Diagnosis	Treatment
Candida albicans, Candida tropicalis	Fever, tachypnoea, tachycardia, organ failure, skin nodules. Meningitis, endophthalmitis, endocarditis	Blood, urine, affected sites such as liver	Amphotericin ± flucytosine. Fluconazole if no neutropenia. Change vascular catheters. Treat any blood isolate
Aspergillus flavus, Aspergillus fumigatus	Pulmonary infiltrates in neutropenic patient, fever. Spreads to any organ	Sputum, bronchoscopy, needle aspiration	Amphotericin
Cryptococcus neoformans	Headache, fever, chest pain cough. Spreads from lungs to CNS and other organs in AIDS or organ transplant	Blood and CSF	Amphotericin or fluconazole
Zygomycetes (Mucormycosis)	Progressive infection of nasopharynx, lung, brain in diabetes or neutropenia	Nasal scraping or biopsy	Amphotericin and early debridement
Histoplasma capsulatum (from North and South America)	Cough, weight loss, fever. Segmental pulmonary infiltrates. Progressive in AIDS with mucosal ulcers, hepatomegaly, meningitis	Blood, marrow, liver, sputum	Itraconazole or amphotericin
Coccidioides immitis (Central and South America, South West USA)	Fever, cough, chest pain, lung infiltrates. Common in transplant patients	BAL, urine if disseminated, skin, bone, CSF	Itraconazole or amphotericin

Table 3
Diagnosis and treatment of systemic fungal infections.

Viral Infections

There had been over 2.5 million cases of AIDS by mid 1993, all continents being affected, Africa accounting for 70%. Heterosexual transmission and spread through intravenous drug use have increased dramatically. Enzyme linked immunosorbent assay (ELISA) is highly sensitive and specific for the detection of anti-HIV antibodies in the serum but must be confirmed by Western blot, immunofluorescence assay or other means. The testing of an unconscious patient is a decision for the individual clinician which he must be able to justify and it should lead to a change in management.

Most admissions to the ICU are the result of opportunistic infections, with *Pneumocystis carinii* in Europe and USA or tuberculosis, diarrhoea or bacteraemia elsewhere. Pneumonia due to Pneumocystis presents with a progressive pneumonitis, fever, sweats, weight loss, cough and breathlessness. Trophozoites fill the alveoli causing hypoxia and shunting and are seen by silver stain of bronchoalveolar lavage. Mortality in the first episode is 10–20%. Tuberculosis as reactivation or primary infection occurs early in AIDS and a third of HIV infected patients exposed to open disease will develop tuberculosis. Infections with *Mycobacterium kansasii* or *M. avium* complex are a feature of immunosuppression. *M. avium* infection presents with fever, night sweats, diarrhoea and weight loss and haematogenous spread to all organs occurs. Bacterial and fungal infections (see above) are more common in AIDS patients than in others. Cytomegalovirus infection is very common and most cases present with retinitis, painless visual loss and blurring. In a study of 153 bacteraemic patients with SIRS, the presence of HIV infection reduced likely survival of an ICU patient by 75%. However, higher mortality is only observed within 6 months of admission.[17] Critically ill patients with HIV infection can survive beyond 12 months if the opportunistic infection is successfully treated.

Viral encephalitis presents with neck rigidity, headache and fever but also conscious level changes, progressing from confusion to stupor, often with focal neurological signs and fits. Herpes encephalitis causes hallucinations and aphasia while Japanese encephalitis is associated with Parkinsonian syndrome. Lumbar puncture is essential, between 10 and 2000 cells/mm^3 being present in CSF, predominantly mononuclear. The CSF protein is raised, particularly IgG, and excess of a specific antibody in CSF over that in serum suggests infection. Acute and convalescent samples are necessary but treatment will have to be given empirically.

Treatment

Antibiotic choice, dosage and policies

The first choice of antibiotic can have a profound effect on the type and susceptibility of pathogens causing infection. Antibiotics are changed in half of bacteraemic patients once the result of blood cultures is available. When ampicillin and gentamicin were used on a neonatal intensive care unit, 93% of Gram negative bacilli isolated were resistant to ampicillin and 57% to cefuroxime. When empirical treatment was changed to cefuroxime and gentamicin, the proportion resistant declined to 60% and 16% respectively with a marked reduction in the isolation of *Klebsiella pneumoniae*.[26] However, the isolation of enterococci increased (Figure 11).

Empirical treatment

In most cases, antibiotic treatment will have to be chosen as a best guess without the benefit of culture results. Once the pathogen is known, treatment should be altered to the agent with the narrowest spectrum in order to reduce the pressure for emergence of resistance (Table 4). Of 294 patients treated empirically for community acquired pneumonia, a single agent was used in 117 (co–amoxiclav, ureidopenicillin, quinolone or cephalosporin), a combination of β-lactam plus aminoglycoside in 123, β-lactam

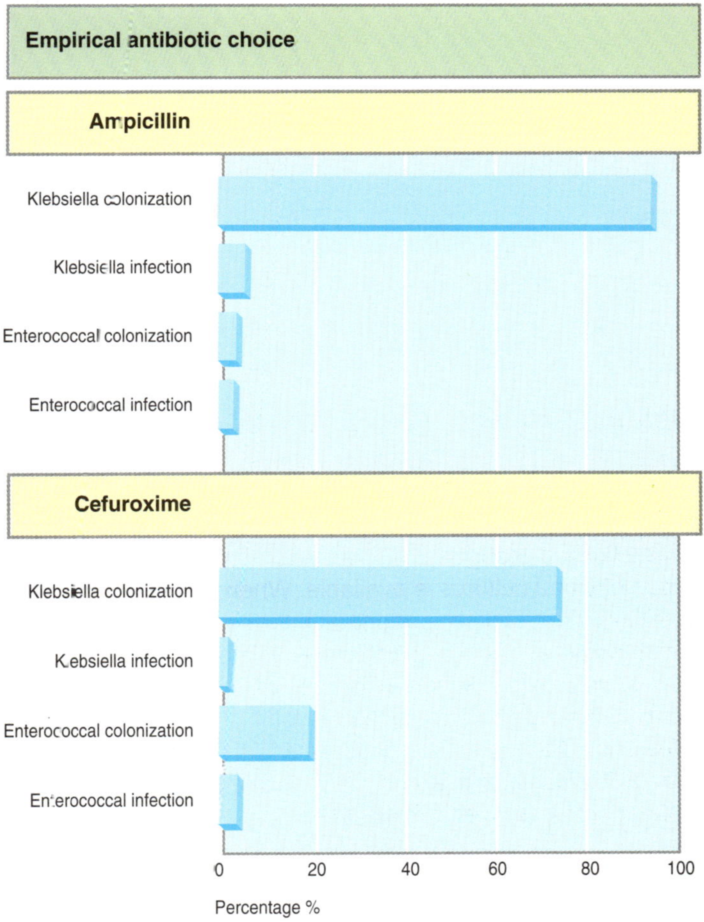

Figure 11
Effect of choice of empirical antibiotic policy on colonization and infection in a neonatal ICU.[26]

plus quinolone in 27, and quinolone plus aminoglycoside in 23.[16] In 92 patients, treatment failed and in 11 of these, the pathogen was resistant to the antibiotic used. A total of 85 (29%) died. Usually, treatment should be reviewed at five days and either stopped or modified according to antibiotic susceptibilities.

Indication	Antibiotic treatment	Comments
Bacteraemia	Cefuroxime, cefotaxime or ceftriaxone	Add gentamicin if hypotensive, metronidazole if anaerobes likely
Abdominal/ pelvic sepsis	Cefuroxime (or similar), metronidazole ± gentamicin or clindamycin + gentamicin	Usually polymicrobial bacteraemia
Febrile neutropenic patient	Ceftazidime, ciprofloxacin or piptazobactam. Second line imipenem or meropenem	Add teicoplanin or vancomycin at 48 hours if no response or earlier if line sepsis If chest infiltrates, add amphotericin B (liposomal/colloidal only if renal deterioration or adverse reactions)
Meningitis	Intramuscular penicillin before admission. Cefotaxime or ceftriaxone	Penicillin G remains first choice only for meningococcal disease. Treat for 10–14 days for pneumococcal meningitis, 7–10 days for others
Streptococcus pyogenes	Benzyl penicillin	Immediate high dose treatment
Enterococcal infection	Amoxycillin or azlocillin or piperacillin	Add gentamicin if Gram negative infection possible
VRE	High dose amoxycillin may be effective	Consult microbiologist
MRSA any site	Teicoplanin or vancomycin	Combine with gentamicin or rifampicin if deep sepsis
Community acquired pneumonia		
Lobar	Benzyl penicillin 10 days	Usually pneumococcal. Penicillin can reach high lung concentrations
Bilateral/ segmental	Erythromycin	Atypical infection usually in outbreaks
Any	Cefuroxime + erythromycin	British Thoracic Society recommendation
Nosocomial pneumonia		
<2–3 days ventilated	Cefuroxime, cefotaxime or ceftriaxone 5 days	*S. pneumoniae, Haemophilus influenzae*, coliforms

Indication	Antibiotic treatment	Comments
>3 days ventilated	Ceftazidime, ciprofloxacin or piptazobactam. 5 days	*Pseudomonas aeruginosa*, β-lactamase producing coliforms
Aspiration pneumonia	Clindamycin or cefuroxime plus metronidazole	Anaerobes and upper respiratory flora
Staphylococcal pneumonia	Clindamycin or flucloxacillin+fusidic acid	Use vancomycin or teicoplanin if MRSA
Legionnaire's disease	Erythromycin (up to 4g/day) + rifampicin 2–3 weeks	Unresponsive to cefuroxime. Associated with organ failure
Pneumocystis pneumonia	Co-trimoxazole or pentamidine or clindamycin plus primaquine	Commonest presentation of AIDS. Adverse reactions frequent
Catheter associated urinary infection	Only if bacteraemic: ceftazidime or ciprofloxacin	*Pseudomonas aeruginosa, Klebsiella* spp, *Enterobacter* spp
Pyelonephritis	Cefuroxime or similar	Add gentamicin if shocked
Diarrhoea	Withdraw antibiotics	Oral vancomycin or oral metronidazole if severe
Cellulitis	Flucloxacillin or nafcillin	High doses will treat both staphylococci and streptococci
Necrotizing fasciitis / gas gangrene	Debridement, benzyl penicillin + metronidazole	High doses and immediate surgery
Bronchiolitis	Supportive	Ribavirin no benefit in older children. Aerosol can be used in infants with cardiac defects
Chickenpox pneumonia	Supportive. Acyclovir in early stages.	Source isolate, only immune staff to attend
Viral encephalitis	Acyclovir	Prolonged supportive treatment
Cytomegalovirus infection	Ganciclovir	Usually AIDS or immune suppressed

Table 4
Empirical and specific treatment of systemic infections.

Gentamicin is a common first line antibiotic but requires careful monitoring to avoid toxicity and should be stopped as soon as there is a clear response. The glycopeptides, teicoplanin and vancomycin, are often needed to cover possible infection with MRSA, coagulase negative staphylococci, multiresistant enterococci or in patients allergic to penicillins. Teicoplanin has the advantage of bolus dosage and does not require monitoring of serum levels. The recommended dose of ciprofloxacin for pseudomonal pneumonia is now 400mg every 12 hours but scientific evidence suggests 400mg every 8 hours is more appropriate.

Prophylaxis

Cefuroxime with or without metronidazole is a frequent choice for operations where a site with a normal flora is entered or in clean surgery where infection is a grave complication. In cardiac surgery, flucloxacillin plus an aminoglycoside is commonly used, although cephalosporins are also effective despite the resistance of most coagulase negative staphylococci. Vancomycin can cause hypotension and teicoplanin may not achieve sufficiently high tissue levels after a single preoperative dose. Whatever the site, prophylaxis must be given at the start of the operation and there is rarely any justification for prolonging prophylaxis for more than 24 hours.

Selective decontamination

Colonization of the oropharynx by Gram negative aerobes commonly precedes nosocomial pneumonia and multiple organ failure. It can be reduced by selective decontamination (SDD). An oral antifungal agent such as amphotericin B and two non-absorbable antibiotics, usually tobramycin and polymyxin B, are given both as an oral paste and to be swallowed. A systemic antibiotic, usually cefotaxime, is used for the first 4–5 days to ensure a rapid reduction in the Gram negative flora, although this might represent treatment of inapparent infection.

Some studies suggest that SDD reduces both nosocomial pneumonia and mortality. However, most were not placebo controlled or blinded and did not allow for the method of prevention of gastric ulceration. Few trials assess the use of topical decontamination alone. Double blind placebo controlled trials show reductions in the number of episodes of pneumonia, urinary infection and sinusitis but usually without significant reduction in mortality or costs.[27] A meta analysis of 22 trials confirmed this impression. The increased costs of antibiotics used in SDD are closely balanced by the reduced costs of treating infection although two studies found costs were increased. Despite the theoretical risks, emergence of resistant bacteria during SDD is either rare or not easily demonstrated. It is possible that resistance was low level or requires a more prolonged period to emerge.

Treatment of renal and liver failure

Organ failure commonly follows septic shock and itself predisposes to infection. Infection should be aggressively treated. Vancomycin, teicoplanin, the aminoglycosides, cephalosporins and penicillins will all accumulate when creatinine clearance falls below 30 ml/min. Vancomycin and aminoglycoside dosage have to be decided on daily serum assays, the dosage interval being increased rather than the unit dose reduced. Antipseudomonal penicillins have to be given at half normal dosage to avoid bleeding tendency. Erythromycin, clindamycin, chloramphenicol, fusidic acid and rifampicin are metabolized in the liver and, although safe in renal failure, should be avoided in liver failure.

Clearance by haemodialysis or haemofiltration depends on the type of machine and the flow rates and frequency. Specific guidance is scanty. Aminoglycoside dosage must be determined by serum assay. The cephalosporins are eliminated slowly but dosage is usually reduced by ≥50%. For example cefotaxime is given at 1g every 24 hours. The glycopeptides need only be given every 3–7 days. Amphotericin B is not dialysable but can be given in normal dosage in complete renal failure. If renal function is present but deteriorating, liposomal or colloidal preparations should be used.

Immunological therapy for infections

Despite the attractive concept of the use of mediator antibodies and antagonists in the treatment of shock, their efficacy in terms of survival has not been established. Clinical trials have not shown a benefit or have provided contradictory results, some apparently of benefit in shocked patients and others only in the absence of shock. The main disadvantage in their use is the difficulty in identifying the patients who may benefit and those who might be disadvantaged.

Anti–endotoxin monoclonal antibody (HA1A) used in patients with sepsis syndrome results in some early reduction in mortality but there is no significant effect by 28 days. Following an early trial in which subgroup analysis suggested a possible benefit in bacteraemic patients, HA1A was licensed for use in Europe but not in the USA. However, the cost was high ($4000 /dose) and its actual efficacy uncertain resulting in many hospitals restricting its use. A second randomized double blind trial was halted when an interim analysis of patients suggested higher mortality in treated patients without bacteraemia and no advantage in Gram negative bacteraemia.[28] Of 621 patients entered, 14 day mortality was 33% in those given the antibody and 32% in those given placebo. For patients without Gram negative bacteraemia, the rates were 41% and 37% ($p=0.07$). The agent was withdrawn in January 1993. The E5 anti-endotoxin antibody improved recovery from organ failure but not survival (Figure 12).[29]

Anti–TNF antibodies in animals prevent death following Gram negative bacteraemia or staphylococcal septicaemia and in patients, high serum TNF concentrations have been associated with greater mortality. TNF and IL–6 concentrations decrease significantly in patients who survive septic shock. However,

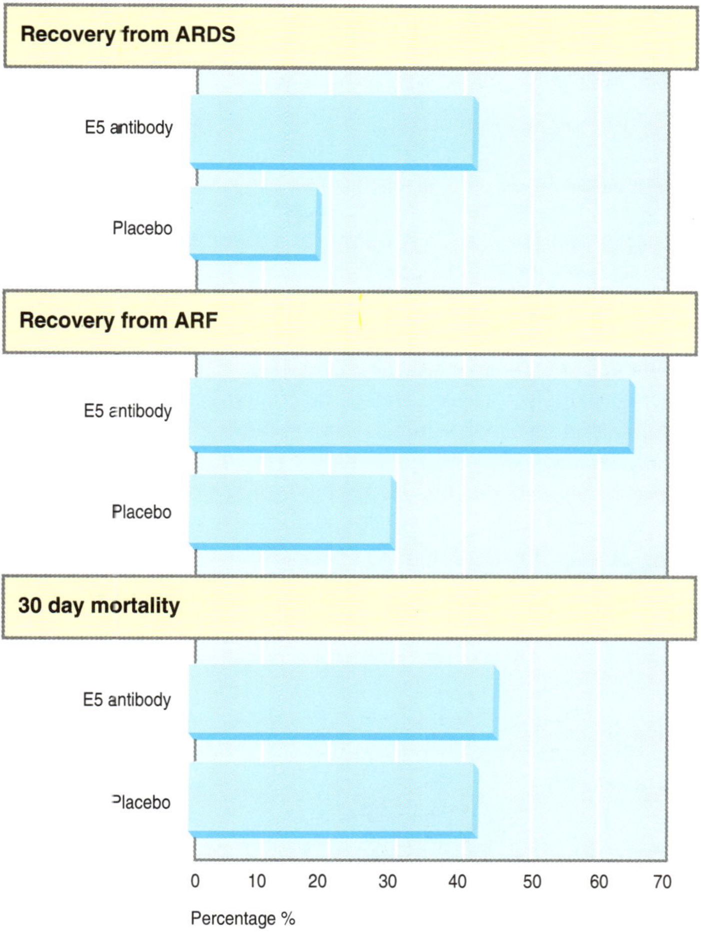

Figure 12
Outcome of administration of E5 monoclonal antibody to endotoxin (ARF = acute renal failure).[29]

no improvement in 28 day survival was found in 80 patients given a murine anti–TNFα antibody and most developed antibodies against the agent. Another trial of 800 patients showed no benefit in patients without shock but at high doses there was a trend to improved survival in shocked patients.[30]

Of 994 patients in a third trial 28 day mortality was 46% in the placebo group, and 38% in the treated group. It is not possible to reliably predict which patients might benefit from anti–TNF therapy but the greatest benefit is only likely to be achieved when it is given at the onset of sepsis.

Interleukin–1 receptor antagonist may increase survival in patients with sepsis or septic shock. Compared with a 44% death rate in a placebo group, only 25% died in a group given 67 mg/hour and 16% in a group having 133 mg/hour.[30] However, a placebo controlled trial of 893 patients in which some patients received 1 or 2 mg/kg/hour found no effect on 28 day mortality. A receptor antagonist to platelet activating factor, another mediator implicated in the inflammatory cascade, has also been tested in clinical trials but only by retrospective sub group analysis could an advantage in mortality be claimed.

Infection in particular patient groups

1. **Cardiac surgery** All patients experience fever for 1–2 days following cardiopulmonary bypass. Thereafter respiratory infection secondary to interstitial oedema is most likely and cefuroxime is appropriate. Infection of the sternal wound usually starts with a serous discharge from the lower end and in a few cases may progress to mediastinitis and dehiscence. *Staphylococcus aureus* or coagulase negative staphylococci (pure or repeated isolates) can be treated with flucloxacillin plus fusidic acid or a glycopeptide but antibiotics are less important than daily dressings. Prosthetic valve endocarditis can present at 1–2 weeks with fever being the only sign causing confusion with the benign post–cardiotomy syndrome. Blood culture is essential.

2. **Gynaecology and obstetrics** Vaginal flora is affected by hospitalization and perioperative antibiotics with the Enterobacteriaceae, *Bacteroides fragilis* and enterococci becoming more common. The duration of surgery, the presence of bacterial vaginosis and site of incision are common risk factors. Fever and pelvic pain 2–3 days after hysterectomy suggest pelvic cellulitis. Blood cultures are essential but the interpretation of samples from the vaginal cuff is difficult. An adnexal abscess can develop several weeks after surgery and is suggested by a swinging fever,

leucocytosis and a palpable mass in the pelvis. Ultrasound will confirm the diagnosis. Clindamycin plus gentamicin or cefuroxime plus metronidazole or co–amoxiclav can be used. Pus rather than swabs must be sent to the laboratory if surgery is performed.

3. **AIDS and Hepatitis** Hepatitis B surface antigen in blood indicates current infection or carriage but transmission is most likely in the presence of the e antigen and/or absence of antibody to the e antigen. Patients from tropical Africa and the Far East, homosexual men, intravenous drug abusers, and cases of acute hepatitis should be considered high risk along with their partners and children. Sufferers need not be source isolated unless the infection is acute, diagnosis is not confirmed or the patient is a Hepatitis e carrier and has open wounds. In patients infected with human immunodeficiency virus (HIV), the blood is infectious whether or not antibody to HIV is detectable. Risk groups are similar to those for Hepatitis B and also include haemophiliacs. Those with open wounds, diarrhoea, or infected with *Mycobacterium tuberculosis* should be isolated.

Precautions in caring for HIV or Hepatitis B carriers

- Staff should wear a plastic apron and gloves for invasive procedures or any contact with body products
- Use a face vizor if splashing is likely
- Bedpans can be disposed in the usual washer (80°C)
- Soiling or blood spills should be cleaned with hypochlorites
- Needles must be disposed in a suitable box without resheathing and linen in a biohazard bag
- Detergent is sufficient for cleaning the room after discharge

Sharps accidents, either inoculation of blood with a contaminated needle or blood splashed into the eyes, are frequent in the ICU raising the possibility of transmission of hepatitis (up to 50%) or HIV (0.3%). All patients, not just known carriers, should be considered potential risks. Staff will in most cases have previously had Hepatitis B vaccine but such injuries should be reported to Occupational Health and the donor screened if necessary, usually with permission. The wound must be washed and blood taken from the recipient to be saved. Hepatitis B vaccine or hyperimmune globulin may be offered if appropriate. The use of zidovudine to prevent HIV seroconversion is unproven, carries a risk of adverse effects and has to be given immediately.

4. **Tuberculosis** The prevalence of tuberculosis has increased in the last ten years partly as the result of reactivation and transmission from patients infected with HIV. Multidrug resistant tuberculosis has emerged through poor compliance with treatment and poses a risk to health workers. Examination of sputum, gastric aspirates or bronchial washing for acid fast bacilli must be made if the diagnosis is suspected following chest X ray. Culture usually takes 4–6 weeks but a radiometric method can give a result in 9–16 days. Isoniazid plus rifampicin for nine months is effective although many advise pyrazinamide plus ethambutol in addition until drug susceptibility is known. Alternatively, the first three agents can be given for two months followed by the first two for four months. Isoniazid, rifampicin and streptomycin can be given by injection in the unconscious patient. In resistant infections, a wide range of other agents may have to be used. Patients newly diagnosed as open tuberculosis must be placed in source isolation for the first 14 days of treatment or longer in the case of resistant organisms.

5. **Burns** The burn wound is initially sterile but soon becomes colonized with *Staphylococcus aureus* in the first week and *Pseudomonas aeruginosa, Acinetobacter* spp and other

Gram negatives in the second. Fever is common irrespective of underlying infection and treatment often has to be given on the basis of cardiovascular instability. The choice of antibiotics should be based on culture results from the wound and blood. Flucloxacillin plus gentamicin in high doses, ciprofloxacin or ceftazidime are popular. Patients should be kept in source isolation as they are efficient disseminators of colonizing agents such as MRSA, especially during dressing changes.

6. **Meningitis and meningococcaemia** Bacterial meningitis is fatal in 10% of cases in children but another 20% suffer hearing loss and up to 10% experience learning difficulties or behaviour disorders. Patients entering the ICU generally require intubation and ventilation. The consumption of plasma components results in bleeding disorders, shock and extravasation. *Neisseria meningitidis* is the most common pathogen in children and young adults while *Streptococcus pneumoniae* is likely in the very young and the old (Figure 13). *Haemophilus influenzae* meningitis in young children has declined with the advent of vaccination. Administration of intramuscular penicillin or chloramphenicol before reaching hospital is recommended and, when available, CT scan of the brain is commonly performed before lumbar puncture to exclude raised intra–cranial pressure. Lumbar puncture will confirm the diagnosis but is then less likely to demonstrate the pathogen (Figure 14). Latex agglutination tests on CSF may demonstrate the common pathogen except *Neisseria meningitidis* group B. Blood culture before antibiotics is helpful.

   Spread occurs by close contact, direct inoculation of mucous membranes or through the respiratory tract. The patient should be source isolated if meningococcal infection is suspected. Rifampicin (or in adults ciprofloxacin) prophylaxis will then be needed for the family contacts and also for siblings in cases of haemophilus meningitis. It is not necessary for hospital staff.

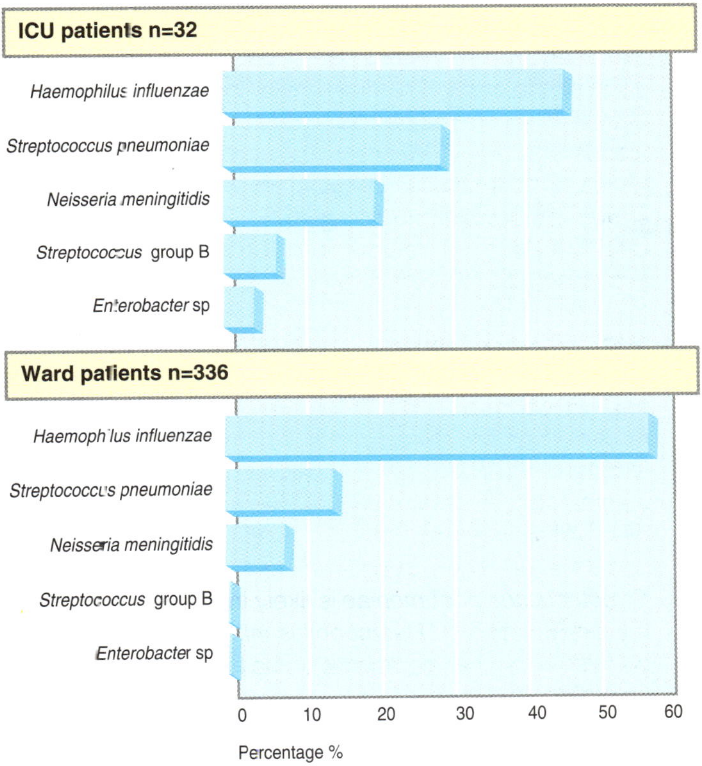

Figure 13
Etiology of bacterial meningitis in children admitted to ICU versus general ward.[31]

Figure 14
Acridine orange stain of CSF showing Neisseria meningitidis. *This stain will demonstrate dead organisms.*

7. **Malaria** Of the species of *Plasmodium* to infect man from the bite of the anopheline mosquito, *P. falciparum* is the most likely to cause disease requiring intensive care. It is frequently resistant to drugs. Diagnosis is by examination of Giemsa–stained blood smear in a patient returned from an endemic area. Continuous fevers, tachycardia, hypotension, cough and headache usually occur in *P. falciparum* infections. Cerebral malaria (seizures and coma), renal failure, hypoglycaemia and anaemia are common complications of a high parasitaemia. Advice from an infectious disease physician must be sought. Chloroquine should not be given. Quinine is given intravenously until the patient can take tablets to finish a seven day course. Tetracycline or fansidar should be used after the quinine. Skilled management of fluids is needed.

8. **Tetanus** Occurring in about 18 per 100 000 population, tetanus is most common in neonates in the developing countries. *Clostridium tetani* is an anaerobic bacillus that produces tetanospasmin during growth which prevents transmitter release from GABAergic neurons. Unrestrained motor neurone activity produces the characteristic spasms in response to stimuli. Trismus, risus sardonicus and abdominal rigidity are followed by generalized spasm. Autonomic dysfunction is the usual cause of death. Neonatal tetanus presents with generalized weakness before the onset of spasms. The illness lasts two weeks and recovery one month. Wound cultures are usually negative. Maintenance of the airway is essential and intubation is usually required. Diazepam and lorazepam antagonize the toxin. Passive immunization with human tetanus immunoglobulin will shorten the disease. The role of penicillin or metronidazole is controversial and surgical attention to the wound can await control of the spasms.

9. **Viral haemorrhagic fevers** Lassa fever is acquired from infected rat urine only in parts of West Africa and sub clinical infections are common. Marburg disease and Ebola

are rare potentially fatal infections usually contracted in central Africa. Congo–Crimean haemorrhagic fever and similar viruses are spread by tick bite or infected blood. Transmission is likely through needlestick injury or contact of blood with open wounds or close contact with pulmonary disease. In patients returning from endemic countries, particularly after travel out of the cities, fever, sore throat, diarrhoea, bleeding into mucous membranes and skin and a rash should suggest the diagnosis. The patient should be source isolated, staff access kept to a minimum and a list of contacts kept. Further action depends on discussion with infectious disease, communicable disease and microbiology consultants. Transfer to a Regional Isolation Unit and follow up of contacts may be necessary.

References

1. Taylor LJ. Health Service Research Concerted Action. Nosocomial Infection Survey.EURO.NIS European Community COMAC, London. (Personal communication).

2. Sproat LJ, Inglis TJJ. A multicentre survey of hand hygiene practice in intensive care units. *J Hosp Infect* 1994; **26**: 137–48.

3. Bauer TM, Ofner E, Just HM, Just H, Daschner FD. An epidemiological study assessing the relative importance of airborne and direct contact transmission of microorganisms in a medical intensive care unit. *J Hosp Infect* 1990;**15**: 301–9.

4. Zimakoff J, Stormark M, Larsen SO. Use of gloves and handwashing behaviour among health care workers in intensive care units. A multicentre investigation in four hospitals in Denmark and Norway. *J Hosp Infect* 1993; **24**: 63–7.

5. Guidelines/Practice Parameters Committee of the American College of Critical Care Medicine, Society of Critical Care Medicine. Guidelines for intensive care unit design. *Crit Care Med* 1995; **23**: 582–8.

6. Huebner J, Frank U, Kappstien I, Just HM, Noeldge G, Geiger K, Daschner FD. Influence of architectural design on nosocomial infections in intensive care units - a prospective 2–year analysis. *Intensive Care Med* 1989; **15**: 179–83.

7. Casewell M, Phillips I. Hands as route of transmission for Klebsiella species. *BMJ* 1977; **2**: 1315–17.

8. Fassbender K, Pargger H, Muller W, Zimmerli W. Interleukin-6 and acute phase protein concentrations in surgical intensive care unit patients: Diagnostic signs in nosocomial infection. *Crit Care Med* 1993; **21**: 1175–80.

9. Pittet D, Rangel–Frausto S, Li N, Tarara D, Costigan M, Rempe L, Jebson P, Wenzel RP. Systemic inflammatory response syndrome, sepsis, severe sepsis and septic shock: incidence, morbidities and outcomes in surgical ICU patients. *Intensive Care Med* 1995; **21**: 302–9.

10. Griffin J, Meduri GU. Diagnosis of nosocomial pneumonia: new approaches. *Med Clin North Am* 1994; **78**: 1091–22.

11. Estes RJ, Meduri GU. The pathogenesis of ventilator associated pneumonia: I. Mechanisms of bacterial transcolonization and airway inoculation. *Intensive Care Med* 1995; **21**: 365–83.

12. Bonten MJM, Gaillard CA, Wouters EFM, van Tiel FH, Stobberingh EE, van der Geest S. Problems in diagnosing nosocomial pneumonia in mechanically ventilated patients: A review. *Crit Care Med* 1994; **22**: 1683–91.

13. Salata RA, Lederman MM, Schlaes DM et al. Diagnosis of nosocomial pneumonia in intubated, intensive care unit patients. *Am Rev Respir Dis* 1987; **135**:426–32.

14. Cook DJ, Brun–Buisson C, Guyatt GH, Sibbald WJ. Evaluation of new diagnostic technologies: bronchoalveolar lavage and the diagnosis of ventilator associated pneumonia. *Crit Care Med* 1994; **22**: 1314–22.

15. Pugin J, Auckenthaler R, Mili N et al. Diagnosis of ventilator associated pneumonia by bacteriologic analysis of bronchoscopic and non-bronchoscopic "blind" bronchoalveolar lavage fluid. *Am Rev Resp Dis* 1991; **143**: 1121–29.

16. Leroy O, Santré C, Beuscart C, Georges H, Guery B, Jacquire JM, Beaucaire G.A five year study of severe community-acquired pneumonia with emphasis on prognosis in patients admitted to an intensive care unit. *Intensive Care Med* 1995; **21**: 24–31.

17. Shoemaker WC, Appel PL, Kram HB, Bishop MH, Abraham E. Sequence of physiologic patterns in surgical septic shock. *Crit Care Med* 1993; **21**:1876–89.

18. Sasse KC, Nauenberg E, Long A, Anton B, Tucker HJ, Hu T. Long term survival after intensive care unit admission with sepsis. *Crit Care Med* 1995; **23**:1040–47.

19. Rello J, Ricart M, Mirelis B, Quintana E, Gurgui M, Net A, Prats G. Nosocomial bacteremia in a medical – surgical intensive care unit: epidemiologic characteristics and factors influencing mortality in 111 episodes. *Intensive Care Med* 1994; **20:** 94–8.

20. Bone RC. Sepsis and its complications: The clinical problem. *Crit Care Med* 1994; **22**: S8–S11.

21. Knaus WA, Harrell FE, Fisher CJ et al. The clinical evaluation of new drugs for sepsis. A prospective study design based on survival analysis. *JAMA* 1993; **270**: 1233–41.

22. Elliott TSJ, Faroqui MH, Armstrong RF, Hanson GC. Guidelines for good practice in central venous catheterization. *J Hosp Infect* 1994; **28**: 163–76.

23. Maki DG, Stolz SS, Wheeler S, Mermel LA. A prospective, randomized trial of gauze and two polyurethane dressings for site care of pulmonary artery catheters: Implications for catheter management. *Crit Care Med* 1994; **22**: 1729–37.

24. Collignon P, Soni N, Pearson I, Sorrell T et al. Sepsis associated with central vein catheters in critically ill patients. *Intensive Care Med* 1988; **14**: 227–31.

25. Conly JM, Grieves K, Peters B. A prospective, randomized study comparing transparent and dry gauze dressings for central venous catheters. *J Infect Dis* 1989; **159**: 310–19.

26. Kalenic S, Francetic I, Polak J, Zele – Starcevic L, Bencic Z. Impact of ampicillinand cefuroxime on bacterial colonization and infection in patients on a neonatal intensive care unit. *J Hosp Infect* 1993; **23**: 35–41.

27. Silver MR, Bone RC. Selective digestive decontamination in critically ill patients.*Crit Care Med* 1993; **21**: 1418–19.

28. Brun–Buisson C. The HA 1A saga: the scientific and ethical dilemma of innovative and costly therapies. *Intensive Care Med* 1994; **20**: 314–6.

29. Bone RC, Balk RA, Fein AM et al. A second large controlled clinical study of E5 a monoclonal antibody to endotoxin: Results of a prospective, multicenter randomized controlled trial. *Crit Care Med* 1995; **23**: 994–1006.

30. Suffredini AF. Current prospects for the treatment of clinical sepsis. *Crit Care Med* 1994; **22**: S12–S18.

31. Madagame ET, Havens PL, Bresnahan JM, Babel KL, Splaingard ML. Survival and functional outcome of children requiring mechanical ventilation during therapy for acute bacterial meningitis. *Crit Care Med* 1995; **23**: 1279–1283.

Index

Page numbers in *italic* refer to the illustrations